GW00367523

Man
Mini Manual

Contents

© Ian Banks 2010   *(12465/007)*
Revision due March 2012

ISBN 978 1 906121 63 1

Printed by J. H. Haynes & Co. Ltd., Sparkford, Yeovil, Somerset BA22 7JJ, England.

Haynes Publishing
Sparkford, Yeovil, Somerset BA22 7JJ, England

Haynes North America, Inc
861 Lawrence Drive, Newbury Park, California 91320, USA

Haynes Publishing Nordiska AB
Box 1504, 751 45 UPPSALA, Sweden

How to get the best from your GP

Write down your symptoms before you see your doctor

- It is easy to forget the most important things during the examination. Doctors home-in on important clues. When did it start? How did it feel? Did anyone else suffer as well? Did this ever happen before?

Arrive informed

- Check out the net for information before you go to the surgery.

Ask questions

- Don't be afraid to ask questions about what a test will show, how a particular treatment works, and when you should come back. After all, it's your man machine.

Avoid asking for night visits unless there is a good reason

- Calling your GP after you have 'suffered' all day at work will antagonise a doctor who thinks personal health should come before convenience.

Don't beat around the bush

- If you have a lump on your testicles say so. With an average of only seven minutes for each consultation its important to get to the point.

Listen to what the doctor says

- If you don't understand, say so. It helps if they write down the important points. Most people pick up less than half of what their doctor has told them.

Have your prescription explained

- Three items on a scrip will cost you as much as a half decent tyre. Ask whether you can buy any of them from the chemist.

Make sure you know what they are all for. Some medicines clash badly with alcohol.

If you want a second opinion say so

- Ask for a consultant appointment by all means but remember you are dealing with a person with feelings and not a computer. Compliment him for his attention first but then explain your deep anxiety.

Be courteous with all the staff

- Receptionists are not dragons trying to prevent you seeing a doctor. Practice nurses increasingly influence your treatment. General practice is a team effort and you will get the best out of it by treating all its members with respect.

Trust your doctor

- There is a difference between trust and blind faith. Your health is a partnership between you and your doctor where you are the majority stakeholder.

Change your GP with caution

- Thousands of people change their doctor each year. Most of them have simply moved house. You do not need to tell your family doctor if you wish to leave their practice. Your new doctor will arrange for all your notes to be transferred. The whole point of general practice is to build up a personal insight into the health of you and your family. A new doctor has to start almost from scratch.

Don't be afraid to ask to see your notes

- You have the right to see what your doctor writes about you.

Depression

Introduction

There are basically two types of depression, both of which can be helped in different ways. It is entirely normal to react with sadness to personal loss. This kind of sadness reaction caused by something external to the person is said to be 'exogenous' or 'reactive depression'.

Depression becomes abnormal when it occurs without an apparent external cause, or when its duration and intensity are out of all proportion to any external cause. This is 'endogenous depression'.

Symptoms

Clinical depression involves a high degree of hopeless despondency, dejection, fear and irritability. Such a degree of sadness in clinical depression is out of all proportion to any external cause. Often there are symptoms such as:

a) *a general slowing down of body and mind.*
b) *insomnia with early morning waking.*
c) *mood worse in the morning.*
d) *slow speech, poor concentration.*
e) *in some cases, restlessness and agitation.*

There are also other psychological symptoms, such as:

a) *confusion.*
b) *self-reproach.*
c) *self-accusation.*
d) *loss of self-esteem.*
e) *loss of sexual interest.*
f) *loss of appetite.*

Causes

Whilst there are known biochemical changes in the brain associated with depression, it is not clear how these come about. There is a great deal of evidence that by modifying these chemical changes depression can be relieved.

The development of antidepressant drugs (see below) has brought this information to light.

Diagnosis

Clinical depression is diagnosed by an interview with the affected person in which it becomes clear that there is a definite mood disorder out of all proportion to any known cause.

Treatment

Effective antidepressant drugs are available, with complex names such as monoamine oxidase inhibitors, tricyclics, and serotonin re-uptake inhibitors, but the treatment of depression involves more than just prescribing drugs. Skilled investigation of the problem, management and advice can be just as important as drug treatment.

Action

Make an appointment to see your GP or ring the Samaritans (08457 90 90 90).

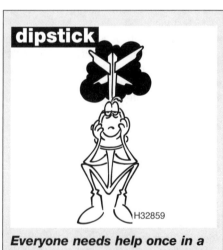

dipstick

H32859

Everyone needs help once in a while. If you're feeling lost don't be afraid to ask for directions

Weight

More than half of us men are overweight – and the proportion is increasing by about one per cent a year. B

Why bother to lose weight?

You'll feel better. As you're able to exert greater control over your body size and shape:

a) *Your self-esteem and self-confidence will rise.*

b) *You'll have more energy.*

c) *Your penis could start to look longer.*

d) *Your sex drive will increase.*

e) *You'll snore less.*

f) *You'll live longer.*

The fat facts

- Lighter men live longer on average. A man of any age who weighs 11.5 stone and is 5 feet 10 inches tall has a 30% lower risk of dying in any given year than a man of the same height who weighs 16.5 stone.
- Non-obese men generally have healthier hearts. A 20% rise in body weight creates an 86% greater risk of heart disease.
- Losing weight can lower blood pressure.
- Obese men are more likely to develop cancer.
- Being overweight increases the risk of arthritis.

Are you overweight?

There are three easy ways of working out whether your health could be at risk.

The waist test

Your circumference is a good, rough-and-ready indicator of your overall body fat level. Simply stand up and find your natural waist line (it's mid-way between your lowest rib and the top of the hip bone). Place a tape around this line and take a measurement after relaxing your abdomen by breathing out gently. If you measure 37-39.5 inches, you're technically overweight. If your waist tops 40 inches, then you're clinically obese.

The body mass index

To calculate your body mass index (BMI): *Multiply your weight in pounds by 700 and divide that figure by the square of your height in inches. For example, if you're 68 inches tall and weigh 185 lb, your BMI = 185 x 700 ÷ (68 x 68 = 4624) = 28.*

Ideally, your score should be between 20 and 25 (in fact, a BMI of about 22 is probably best for long-term health); below 20 and you're underweight; between 25 and 30, you're overweight; and if you're above 30, you're obese. This is the standard test used to check whether your weight could cause health problems. It's not so suitable for fit men with loads of muscle, however, since they could seem overweight even though they're actually carrying very little fat.

The waist : hip ratio

Measure your waist and hips. (It doesn't matter whether you do this in centimetres or inches.) Measure the circumference of your waist as described in the waist test; your hips should be measured at their widest part.

Divide your waist measurement by your hip measurement to get a ratio. For example, if your waist is 35.5 inches and your hips 41 inches, the ratio is 0.86. If your ratio is greater than 0.95, you need to lose some weight. This is a particularly useful test because it assesses your fat distribution and calculates whether you have too much around your abdomen.

Diabetes

Introduction

Sugar in the blood varies between certain fairly narrow limits. Because people with diabetes have little or no insulin (a hormone that breaks down sugar), there is a constant tendency for the blood sugar levels to rise. An excessive rise is associated with the over-production of dangerous acidic substances called 'ketones'.

Type I or insulin dependent diabetes, in which the man produces no insulin, affects about 1% of the population.

Type II diabetes, often called maturity-onset diabetes, is regarded as a condition in which the body cells don't react to insulin, or in which the amount of insulin produced by the pancreas is not enough for the body to function normally.

Symptoms

Thirst, excessive urine and in type I diabetes, weight loss are the major symptoms.

Causes

Diabetes is caused by the failure of the specialised pancreas cells called islet cells to produce the hormone insulin. Insulin is essential for the building up of important large molecules, such as fats, proteins and glycogen, from small molecules such as glucose and amino acids and for the uptake of glucose for energy by cells such as muscle cells.

Diagnosis

Diabetes is diagnosed by finding sugar in the urine, and by testing the levels of blood sugar at different times of day.

Prevention

At present it is not possible to prevent type I diabetes.

The risk of type II diabetes can be greatly reduced by eating less so as to avoid obesity.

Treatment

Type I diabetes is treated with insulin injections and diet and exercise control, all monitored by frequent checks of the blood sugar levels.

Type II diabetes is treated by weight loss, diet control, oral hypoglycaemic drugs and also insulin injections.

Action

Make an appointment to see your GP.

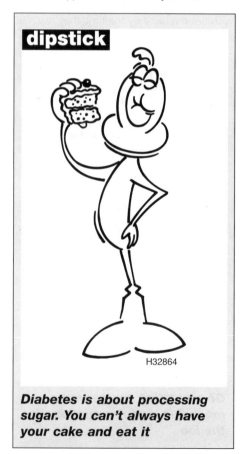

dipstick

H32864

Diabetes is about processing sugar. You can't always have your cake and eat it

Prostate problems

Introduction

Sitting at the neck of the bladder, the prostate is roughly the size of a walnut and has an important job of providing nutrients and protection for the sperm about to make the long journey to the womb. Should the prostate enlarge too much it can obstruct the flow of urine from the bladder to the penis. When this is caused by simple enlargement with no involvement of cancer, it is referred to as Benign Prostatic Hypertrophy (BPH). Over 30% of men will have some problem with passing urine by the time they reach 50 years of age.

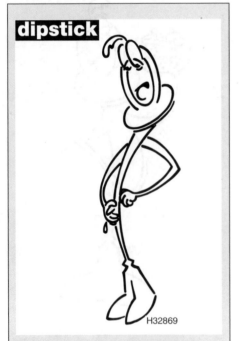

dipstick

H32869

Go and speak to your man mechanic if you're misfiring in the loo

Symptoms

Poor urinary flow; frequent trips to the toilet even during the night. A persistent feeling of 'not quite emptying the bladder' often with dribbling after passing urine.

Causes

We don't know why it enlarges but there are certain triggers:
- a) *High levels of testosterone, the male sex hormone.*
- b) *An imbalance between oestrogen and testosterone.*
- c) *Possibly, low protein, high carbohydrate diets, high fat diets.*
- d) *Western diets.*

Prevention

Even though we are not sure of the exact cause of either benign prostatic enlargement or prostate cancer, sensible protection would involve:
- a) *Weight reduction if you are overweight.*
- b) *Limit animal fat intake, and reduce all fats anyway.*
- c) *Eat at least half a kilo of fruit per day.*
- d) *Increase your intake of antioxidants by eating carrots and citrus fruits.*

Complications

Urinary retention, being unable to pass water properly, can damage the kidneys.

Action

Make an appointment to see your GP immediately if there is any blood in the urine or sperm.

Prostate Cancer

Introduction

British men have a 1 in 12-lifetime risk of developing prostate cancer, roughly the same as a woman developing breast cancer.

Symptoms

Unfortunately there may be no symptoms until the disease is well advanced. It can also be confused with less dangerous conditions such as an inflammation of the prostate (prostatitis) and a gradual increase in size of the prostate without any cancer present (benign prostatic hypertrophy or BPH).

You may experience:
a) *Poor flow of urine.*
b) *Frequent trips to the toilet.*
c) *A persistent feeling of 'not quite emptying the bladder'.*
d) *Blood in the urine or semen.*
e) *A severe backache.*

Causes

We don't know the exact causes but there may be certain triggers:
a) *High levels of testosterone (the male sex hormone).*
b) *An imbalance between oestrogen and testosterone.*
c) *Western diets.*

Contrary to popular belief, prostate cancer is not restricted to the over 70's but is now becoming more common in the 50 plus age group. There is an increased risk of developing prostate cancer if you have a close family member who has suffered from the condition.

Prevention

There are no hard and fast rules for preventing prostate cancer. Common sense protection might include:

a) *Reduce red meat and animal fat in your diet.*
b) *Avoid being overweight.*
c) *Eat plenty of fruit and vegetables.*

There is great debate over the value of screening for prostate cancer. The best test for prostate cancer is the PSA test which measures the levels of a prostate protein (Prostate Specific Antigen) in the blood. This is only of any real value in men who are experiencing symptoms. But when combined with a Digital Rectal Examination (DRE) (a doctor checking the back passage with a gloved finger), the accuracy of the detection rate of these tests ranges from 80%-90%.

Treatment

Treatment choice generally remains between surgery and radiotherapy. Hormone treatment may also slow down the growth of the cancer. Other treatments are being developed.

Complications

Surgical treatments for prostate cancer can cause erectile dysfunction and incontinence. The cancer itself can cause problems with passing water.

If the cancer spreads to the spine it can cause back pain which can be treated with painkillers and radiotherapy.

Self care

Keeping fit and mentally active is important. Prostate cancer tends to develop very slowly. Life can go on almost as normal.

Action

If you are concerned, make an appointment with your GP.

7

Erectile dysfunction (impotence)

Introduction

Problems with erections are common. More than half of all men over 40 report some form of erectile dysfunction (ED) at some stage of their lives. ED is not the same as infertility. A man can father children without being able to have an erection.

For most cases of ED there will be a varying mixture of psychological and physical causes, along with adverse affects of medicines. Around 20 to 30% of all cases will be purely psychological (resulting from stress or anxiety) and will often respond well to non-clinical treatments such as sex counselling.

Generally speaking, if you have erections at any time other than during attempted intercourse then you are more likely to have a psychological rather than physical problem. Successful erections during television programmes, sexy videos or masturbation bodes well for the future, although it is not a 100% test.

Symptoms

Being unable to establish and / or maintain an erection sufficient for making love is about the best description.

ED usually has a gradual onset.

Causes

The penis works by hydrostatic pressure allowing blood in to the spongy tissues of the penis but restricting its outflow. Anything which affects the arteries, veins or nerves which bring this about will influence the ability to have an erection.

Certain anti depressants can make ED worse and some blood pressure drugs are common culprits.

Alcohol is a common cause. Obviously binge drinking has an immediate effect but chronic alcohol abuse can lead to permanent problems. Small amounts of alcohol in the blood (a couple of drinks) make erections easier. Any more can cause the dreaded 'droop'.

Diseases which affect the nerves or blood supply can also cause problems:
- Multiple sclerosis can cause ED.
- Diabetes can damage nerves, which affect the ability to have an erection.
- Problems with blood circulation account for around 25% of ED in men.

dipstick

H32855

Not firing on all cylinders? Get to your man mechanic for a check-up

Prevention

Avoiding excessive alcohol is the obvious first line to preventing 'droop'. Unfortunately erection problems can be much more serious than that. It's all about blood flow, and some pretty simple mechanics, so keeping your cardiovascular system healthy is important. You know the drill, don't smoke, don't drink too much.

Check with your doctor whether any drugs you are taking could be part of the problem.

Treatment

If you think you've got a problem, get in to see your doctor. Yes it's embarrassing, but let's face it, the doctor really has seen it all before. Try to keep it business-like to prevent embarrassment. Bring along a checklist of questions to ask, and think about answers to these common questions ready:

● Are you currently drinking heavily or finding yourself under heavy stress?
● When was the last time you successfully had sexual intercourse?
● Do you wake up with an erection (so called 'morning glory')?

However, it's not just about the doctor asking you questions. ED can seriously affect

who you are. So think about how different treatments might affect your normal sex life.

Remember that in the majority of cases ED can be effectively treated, and by working with your GP you will get the best treatment. Your doctor is no mind reader, so if he gives you a treatment and it doesn't work (give it some time though, some treatments need a few goes for best results), you are quite within your rights to go back and tell him. There may be other treatments that can be tried.

Vacuum devices have been around for over 70 years. They work by drawing blood into the penis under a gentle vacuum produced by a sheath placed over the penis and evacuated with a small pump. By restricting the blood from leaving with a tight rubber band at the base of the penis, a respectable erection can be produced. It makes sense to remove the band after 30 minutes or so to avoid problems with blood clotting. They can be used in men with vascular problems.

More recently oral treatments have been developed which, for some, are more convenient than devices or injections. Its important to discuss these with your doctor as some work differently to others; some work better in certain men, and some have important interactions with other medicines (particularly nitrates for relief from angina). Talk to your doctor about which might be best for you. If it doesn't work, tell him, and ask to try an alternative or a higher dose.

Remember too, oral treatments will not increase your sex drive.

Injections of medicine straight into the penis will produce an erection in virtually all men, with or without sexual stimulation. The needle is so fine it is virtually painless but you need to inject into different places to stop any scarring.

Herbal and traditional remedies are freely available but there is little evidence that they work. Most contain yohimbine, a bark extract which at best can only be described as marginally useful.

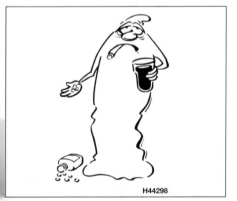

H44298

Medicines and alcohol can be a factor

Testicular cancer

Introduction

Thankfully testicular problems are relatively rare. Testicular cancer is the most serious. It represents only 1% of all cancers in men, but it is the single biggest cause of cancer related death in men aged between 18 and 35 years although it can develop in boys as young as 15. Currently about 1500 men a year develop the disease. Unfortunately the number of cases has doubled in the last 20 years and is still rising.

Symptoms

- A lump on one testicle.
- Pain and tenderness in either testicle.
- Discharge (pus or smelly goo) from the penis.
- Blood in the sperm at ejaculation.
- A build up of fluid inside the scrotum.
- A heavy dragging feeling in the groin or scrotum.
- An increase in size of the testicle. (It is normal for one testicle to be larger then the other, but the sizes and shape should remain more or less the same.)
- An enlargement of the breasts, with or without tenderness.

Causes

The causes of the increase are unknown. Exposure to female hormones in the environment, in water (possibly from the oral contraceptive pill in water supplies), or in baby milk have been suggested. In Spain and most Asian countries there has been no significant increase but we do not know why. At the same time sperm counts are falling across Europe and this may be part of the picture. Undescended testicles are a major factor (where the testicle stays inside the body after birth and will not sit in

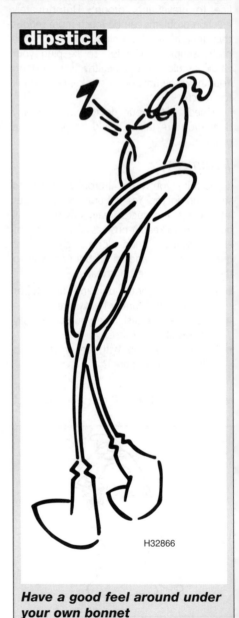

dipstick

H32866

Have a good feel around under your own bonnet

the scrotum). Men with one or two undescended testes have a greatly increased risk – one in 44. The condition can be corrected surgically, but must be done before the age of 10.

Your risk increases if your father or brother suffered from testicular cancer.

Prevention

For once men are positively encouraged to feel themselves, but this time to do more

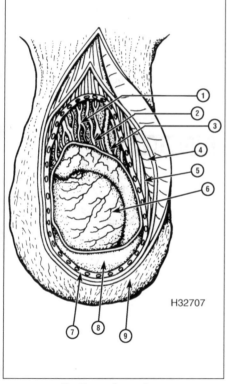

Testis and scrotum

1	Vein	6	Testis
2	Artery	7	Muscle
3	Vas deferens	8	Tunica vaginalis
4	Epididymis	9	Skin
5	Fascia		

H32707

than 'check they're still there'. Self examination is the name of the game. Check your tackle monthly like this:

Do it lying in a warm bath or while having a long shower, as this makes the skin of the scrotum softer and easier therefore, to feel the testicles inside.

Cradle the scrotum in the palm of your hand. Feel the difference between the testicles. You will almost definitely feel that one is larger and lying lower. This is completely normal.

Examine each one in turn, and then compare them with each other. Use both hands and gently roll each testicle between thumb and forefinger. Check for any lumps or swellings as they should both be smooth. Remember that the duct carrying sperm to the penis, the epididymis, normally feels bumpy. It lies along the top and back of the testis.

Complications

Many types of testicular cancer can be cured in around 96% of cases if caught at an early stage. Even when these tumours spread, they can still be cured in 80% of cases, and large volume tumours can be cured in 60% of cases. Even so, late diagnosis increases the risk of a poorer response to treatment.

One testicle may need to be removed, but a prosthesis (false one) disguises the fact almost completely.

Treatment with radiotherapy or radiography may affect your ability to father children, but in many cases fertility is not affected. It is also possible to store sperm before treatment.

Self care

Too frequent self examination can actually make it more difficult to notice any difference and may cause unnecessary worry.

Heart attack

Introduction

An acute myocardial infarction (heart attack) is what happens when the blood supply to a part of the heart muscle has been cut off by blockage of one of the coronary arteries.

When blood is restricted or cut off the cells start to die.

Heart attack is the final result of a disease of the heart arteries (coronary artery disease) called atherosclerosis. About five people in every 1000, mostly men, suffer a heart attack in the UK each year.

Symptoms

A heart attack can involve:
a) *Crushing central chest pain (often described as a 'vice around the chest').*
b) *Breathlessness.*
c) *Clammy skin, sweating and pale complexion.*
d) *Dizziness, nausea and vomiting.*
e) *Restlessness.*

The pain often travels to the neck, jaws, ears, arms and wrists. Less often, it travels to between the shoulder blades or to the stomach. The pain does not pass on resting as in angina.

Severe pain is not always present. In less major cases pain may be absent and there is evidence that up to 20% of mild heart attacks are not recognised as such, or even as significant illness, by those affected.

Causes

Blockage of the coronary arteries caused by a clot (thrombosis) from fatty material caught in the blood.

When total blockage occurs, part of the heart muscle loses its blood supply and dies. Depending on the size of the artery blocked, a larger or smaller portion of the heart will be affected.

Risk factors include:
a) *Smoking cigarettes.*
b) *Being overweight.*
c) *Abnormally high blood pressure.*
d) *High blood cholesterol level.*
e) *A diet high in saturated fats (animal fats).*
f) *Diabetes.*
g) *A family history of heart disease.*
h) *Lack of regular exercise.*

Diagnosis

The ECG (electro cardiograph) draws a tracing of the electrical changes occurring in the heart with each beat. It also shows which part of the heart muscle has been damaged.

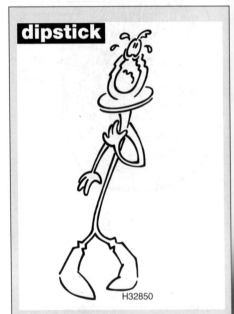

dipstick

H32850

Much worse than a blockage on the M25

A blood test will look for certain heart muscle proteins that are only found in high levels immediately after a heart attack. These are also useful in confirming the diagnosis.

Prevention

The best way to avoid a problem is to stop it happening. Regular body maintenance using the right fuels and getting regular run-outs will help. Here are some pointers:

- Your diet should include a high proportion of fruit and fresh vegetables.
- A small amount of alcohol – such as one glass of wine a day – may be helpful.
- Stop smoking, increase exercise if sedentary and avoid saturated fats.

Complications

Immediate complications are:

a) *Dangerous irregular heart rhythms and very fast or very slow rates.*
b) *Dangerous drops in blood pressure.*
c) *Fluid build-up in and around the lungs.*
d) *Clots forming in the deep veins of the legs or pelvis (deep vein thrombosis).*
e) *Rupture of the heart wall.*

Later complications are:

a) *Ballooning (aneurysm) of the damaged heart wall, which becomes thin and weak.*
b) *Increased risk of another heart attack in the future.*
c) *Angina.*
d) *Poor heart action causing breathlessness and build-up of fluid in the ankles and legs (oedema).*
e) *Depression, loss of confidence, loss of sex drive, and fear of having sex which is common and unfounded.*

Treatment

Cardio-Pulmonary Resuscitation (Kiss of Life).
   Clot-dissolving injections are now routinely used in hospital. These can break down the clot in the coronary artery and allow the damaged heart muscle to recover, sometimes

completely. They must be given within 24 hours at the most. Because the heart rhythm may become temporarily abnormal as it recovers, this treatment is best given when the heart rhythm can be continuously monitored on an ECG. This can be done in an ambulance or in hospital.

In an uncomplicated recovery it is normal to be home within a week or less. Work can be restarted 4–12 weeks after the attack, depending on the level of physical exertion involved with the job. Driving can restart after one month, but DVLA and the motor insurance company must be informed of the heart attack.

Rather than avoiding any exercise it is now known that a return to normal levels of activity – this includes sex – helps prevent any further attacks.

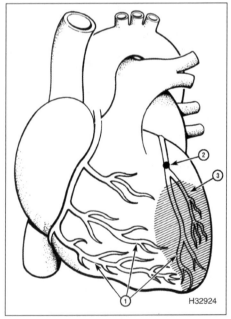

Heart and blood vessels showing what happens in a heart attack

1 *Coronary arteries*   2 *Blockage*
3 *Oxygen starved tissue*

High blood pressure (hypertension)

Introduction

Myths surround every aspect of blood pressure. It helps to know what is being measured in the first place. Blood pressure (BP) is always written as two numbers thus: 120/80. Neither of these numbers has anything to do with your age, height or weight. They are simple measurements of the heart's ability to overcome pressure from an inflated cuff placed around the arm or leg.

As the cuff is slowly deflated, the sound of the blood pushing its way past is suddenly heard in a stethoscope placed over the artery. This is the maximum pressure reached by the heart during its contraction. As the pressure is further released the sound gradually muffles and disappears. This is the lowest pressure in your blood system. Putting the two pressures over each other gives a ratio of the blood pressure while the heart is contracting (systolic) over the pressure while the heart is refilling with blood ready for the next contraction (diastolic). The lower pressure actually represents the pressure caused by the major arteries contracting, keeping the blood moving while the heart refills.

There is no 'normal' blood pressure as it constantly changes within the same person and depends on what they are doing at the time. A blood pressure above 140/90 for anyone at rest should be investigated.

Symptoms

Hypertension is called the silent killer for good reason. Most people do not realise that they are suffering from high blood pressure until something serious happens.

As the pressure steadily rises, damage occurs to the arteries, kidney and heart. For this reason alone it is worth having your blood pressure checked every year or so when you are over the age of 45 years.

There may be some warning signs such as blood in your urine or loss of vision right at the edges (tunnel vision).

Causes

Hypertension can be linked to genetic factors, and this risk is increased by high salt intake, fatty food, obesity, stress, alcohol abuse and lack of activity.

Hypertension can also be caused by other medical conditions, which have an effect on blood pressure. Kidney problems are a good example of this.

Prevention

Just taking a look at the causes will mean that prevention explains itself. Cut down on the salt, reduce your body weight and fat intake, drink alcohol in moderation and stay active. Of all the prevention you can take, exercising three times a week until the point of breathlessness is perhaps the easiest and has the most dramatic effect for decreasing your risk from hypertension.

Complications

Stroke and heart attacks are two of the most common complications from hypertension. It can also damage the kidneys and liver.

Self care

Once diagnosed with hypertension apply all the advice as for prevention. Your doctor may well find that through losing weight increasing activity and reducing alcohol intake you can do without the medication to bring down your blood pressure.

Note

A single reading of blood pressure is unreliable. At least three readings over a few weeks are required. Simply having your blood pressure checked can make it rise in some people (called the white coat effect). Self testing using machines from the pharmacist is a good idea.

Action

Make an appointment to see your GP.

Contacts

British Heart Foundation
14 Fitzhardinge Street,
London W1H 6DH

Diabetes UK
10 Parkway,
London NW1 7AA
Tel: 020 7424 1030

Drinkline
(For advice and information on reducing alcohol consumption)
Tel: 0800 917 8282

McCormack Ltd,
(For TSE Testicular Self Examination Leaflets)
Church House, Church Square,
Leighton Buzzard,
Beds, LU7 7AE.

NHS Direct
(An online health information service includes child health)
Tel: 0845 4647
www.nhsdirect.nhs.uk

Orchid Trust,
Colin Osborne, Chairman,
The Orchid Cancer Appeal,
9 Grace Close,
Hainault, Essex, IG6 3DW.

Prostate Research Campaign UK,
PO Box 2371,
Swindon,
SN1 3LS
Tel 01793 431 901
www.prostate-research.org.uk

Samaritans
(For emotional support for people in crisis or at risk of suicide)
General Office,
10 The Grove,
Slough, Berks SL1 1QP.
Tel: 08457 90 90 90
www.samaritans.org

Stroke Association,
Stroke House,
Whitecross Street,
London EC1Y 8JJ

The Prostate Cancer Charity
3 Angel Walk,
Hammersmith,
London W6 9HX
Tel 0845 300 8383
www.prostate-cancer.org.uk

SELF CARE

You are in charge

Around 7 million UK men live with one or more long term medical conditions. While there may be no cures, effective treatments are accessible. This is your manual – keep it in life's glovebox.

Who, when, where?

Long term medical conditions don't always remain the same. If you think your condition is getting worse, seek advice early rather than wait until an emergency develops. Sources of help include:

Pharmacists – professionals providing advice on the use and selection of prescription and over-the-counter (OTC) medicines. Will tell you if further attention is required.

NHS Walk in Centres – convenient, appointment-free, located in high streets and shopping malls. Highly qualified NHS nurses offer advice, care of minor ailments and injuries, and prescriptions.

NHS Direct – 24 hour confidential health advice and information. Call 0845 4647, or visit NHS Direct online at www.nhsdirect.nhs.uk.

GPs – available from around 8.30 am to 6 pm. There is also an out of hours system. Practices often have minor surgery, skin care and diabetic clinics.

A & E – these hospital departments treat serious accidents or life-threatening illnesses. Open 24/7, they unfortunately tend to be used by people who should really have seen their GP.

Be in charge

People who understand their own medical condition are more likely to take medicines correctly, wind up less often in A & E and be more confident in self care. In other words they are in better control of their lives. If you can, try the 'Expert Patient Programme', where you learn about confidence building, stress, diet, pain, and how to get what you want from health care professionals. National charities also run their own courses. Ask your pharmacist, practice nurse or go onto the web.